FAUCI

EXPECT
THE
UNEXPECTED

FAUCI

EXPECT
THE
UNEXPECTED

Ten Lessons on Truth, Service, and the Way Forward

NATIONAL GEOGRAPHIC

WASHINGTON, D.C.

Since 1888, the National Geographic Society has funded more than 14,000 research, conservation, education, and storytelling projects around the world. National Geographic Partners distributes a portion of the funds it receives from your purchase to National Geographic Society to support programs including the conservation of animals and their habitats.

Get closer to National Geographic Explorers and photographers, and connect with our global community. Join us today at nationalgeographic .com/join

For rights or permissions inquiries, please contact National Geographic Books Subsidiary Rights: bookrights@natgeo.com

Additional quotes and material attributed to Dr. Fauci used by permission.

This title was developed by National Geographic Books in connection with *Fauci,* a National Geographic Documentary Film. It draws from both existing speeches and original interviews given for the film. Dr. Fauci was not paid for his participation and will not earn any royalties from this book's publication or from the documentary.

ISBN: 978-1-4262-2245-0

Printed in the United States of America

21/WOR/1

A LIFE WELL LIVED
IS TO HAVE MADE A
CONTRIBUTION TO
SOCIETY, LEAVING WHAT
YOU'VE TOUCHED BETTER
OFF THAN BEFORE
YOU HAD ANYTHING
TO DO WITH IT.

—DR. ANTHONY FAUCI

CONTENTS

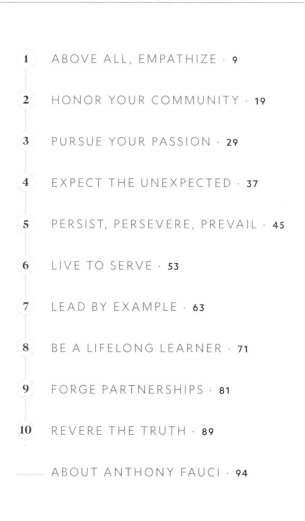

ABOVE ALL, EMPATHIZE

1

. . . .

I ALWAYS TRY TO LOOK FOR
THE POSITIVE IN PEOPLE.
THAT MAY NOT WORK FOR
EVERYBODY, BUT ONE OF MY
GUIDING PRINCIPLES IS EMPATHY.

,

PRIORITIZE PEOPLE

When you're a physician, it's just as important to know human nature as it is to know human physiology. The most important thing in the care of a patient is *caring* for the patient. You've really got to care about them as a person—not as a statistic, or somebody you're going to bill, or somebody who's just one of a number of people.

THERE'S NO GRADATION OF
WHO'S MORE WORTHY OR NOT.

....

FOCUS ON COMPASSION

It's important to empathize with and understand a patient. If you are a physician or another health care provider, you must have nothing less than a complete commitment toward that person and establish a relationship based on sensitivity, comfort, compassion, reassurance, and respect.

Anthony Fauci was almost five years old in 1945 when the United States detonated atomic bombs over the Japanese cities of Hiroshima and Nagasaki, unleashing catastrophic damage and casualties and spurring Japan's surrender to the Allies.

That moment when I saw my mother reading the *New York Daily News* with the big picture on the front page of the devastation in Hiroshima was a memorable moment for me. I had played war games as a child, where the good guys were the GIs and the bad guys were the Japanese, and when I saw the destruction in Japan, I thought, *Wow, hey, that's great.*

But I saw in my mother something that puzzled me at first. Then it became clear that despite the fact that these people were the enemy, my mother had a deep empathy for what they were going through.

I couldn't understand it at the time. I thought, *There're good guys and bad guys. How could you have empathy for the bad guys?* But it got embedded in my mind, and many decades later, I still remember that scene in the living room in our apartment in Brooklyn. I can picture my mother sitting on the couch looking at the paper, and me looking over her knee. She was really sad.

That was a defining moment: understanding that you can feel empathy for people who are very different from you—even people who might officially be the enemy, who are trying to kill you and you're trying to kill them. I saw that you could still feel humanity toward them.

"

TO BE A **GOOD DOCTOR**, OF COURSE YOU'VE GOT TO KNOW WHAT YOU'RE DOING. YOU HAVE TO BE **WELL TRAINED**, AND YOU HAVE TO HAVE A CERTAIN TALENT. YOU CAN'T BE A KLUTZ. YOU'VE GOT TO BE **HUMBLE** ENOUGH, AND **MODEST** ENOUGH, THAT YOU KNOW THAT YOU HAVE TO **KEEP LEARNING**—AND YOU NEED TO KEEP UP WITH THE FIELD. YOU'VE GOT TO HAVE **GOOD JUDGMENT**.

PRACTICE TOLERANCE

Homophobia was clearly pervasive at the outbreak of AIDS. Because I was spending most of my time with sick gay men, I saw homophobia in society—and by association, as their physician, I was on the receiving end of homophobic attacks.

I don't think I ever had any element of homophobia or even any inkling of that in me. I think it gets back to my parents and their tolerance for other people. Empathy was a big component of my growing up in my family—and it was solidified and underscored in Jesuit training in high school and then in college.

I have always felt empathy for people who are being treated unfairly, as well as the unfairness of the prejudice against those whose sexual orientation is part of who they are. The injustice of that has dominated my attitude about what homophobia was and is. It made me angry to see people have that attitude. It made me a defender of others' right to be who they are.

COMBAT STIGMA

During the Obama administration, we needed to remove the stigma from Ebola. That means you don't ostracize the medical personnel who come back from West Africa. You don't ostracize the patients who have recovered from Ebola, because they're not going to hurt anybody. Nina Pham is a nurse who had taken care of an Ebola patient in Dallas and got infected. She was transferred to the National Institutes of Health, where I took care of her, and she recovered well. So when she was getting ready to go back home to Texas, we decided we would publicly discharge her and have a press conference. You can imagine the amount of public interest; it seemed that there were a hundred cameras outside the Clinical Center waiting for her to leave the hospital.

We decided I would go out and say a few words, and then I would introduce Nina. As she came walking toward me, I opened up my arms, threw them around her, and gave her a big hug—which, as you can imagine, went totally viral on social media. I wanted people to see that I was not afraid of hugging someone who had just recovered from Ebola. And then we took her to the White House and introduced her to President Obama, and he hugged her too.

MY OPTIMISM IS THAT THERE ARE
GOING TO BE BAD ACTORS, AND THERE
ARE GOING TO BE BETTER ANGELS.
BUT I THINK THERE ARE MORE BETTER
ANGELS THAN BAD ACTORS.

....

FOCUS OUTWARD

I've tried to instill in my daughters something I think they naturally have just from growing up in our household: a consideration for others. Not to make your life about you but rather about your place in the world and what you can contribute, as well as understanding and dealing with other people—as opposed to an inward-looking attitude of "it's all about me."

SCENE
FROM A
LIFE

was born on Christmas Eve 1940. As my father tells the tale, the obstetrician who was taking my mother through her pregnancy happened to have been at a black-tie cocktail party that night. And when my mother went into labor, apparently it was pretty quick. My father brought her to Brooklyn Hospital, and he remembers the doctor walking in with a tux on. He had to get into the delivery room very quickly, so he just washed his hands and put the scrubs over the tux to deliver me. We always joked about it at home: Just how much had he had to drink before he came in?

HONOR YOUR COMMUNITY

2

THE THING I REMEMBER
ABOUT MY NEIGHBORHOOD
IS ITS WARMTH AND
PROTECTIVE NATURE.

,

DO YOUR PART

We lived above my father's pharmacy. I delivered prescriptions on my bicycle around the neighborhood, and my sister helped out behind the counter. I had a Schwinn bicycle with a basket up front, and I used to do the deliveries for tips. I'd zip around the neighborhood, park my bike, knock on the door, deliver, and they would give me a 25 cent tip. That was a big tip!

I met different people, and I got an appreciation of what illness is—I knew they were ill from the way they looked. That was my first introduction to illness and medicine. And by helping out in the store, I got a better perspective of the family unit because we all worked together.

LOVE IS A LANGUAGE

One of the favorite people in my life was my paternal grandfather. He used to babysit for my sister and me, and he spoke very little English. From the time I was born until the time I went to elementary school, he spoke Italian to me. I can't speak Italian, but he never had to say something twice to me: I knew exactly what he wanted me to do. There were a lot of hand motions with that too.

Fauci spent his early childhood in the Bensonhurst section of Brooklyn, New York, in a neighborhood he describes as 99.9 percent Italian American. All four of his grandparents had immigrated from Italy via Ellis Island, and his parents met and married in New York, moving to Brooklyn from the Lower East Side of Manhattan to raise their family.

I n the summer when the windows were open, the smells were everywhere—mostly tomato sauce and sausages being cooked. And it was something that became part of me. Whenever I happen to smell that now, decades and decades and decades later, it's an immediate flashback. It puts me right back on 79th Street and New Utrecht Avenue, and I can't escape it. There was a certain feeling of freedom, fresh air and sunshine, and being outdoors on the streets of Brooklyn.

It was the safest place in the world to be, because all of the storekeepers sat in their little chairs in front of their shops, watching the kids go by. No one in their wildest dreams would imagine trying to intimidate any of these kids, because the entire neighborhood was kind of like a protective squad. We felt perfectly secure all the time. It was an extremely happy childhood.

THERE'S NO DOUBT THAT THE
IMMIGRANT PHILOSOPHY OF LIFE
PERMEATED MANY OF THE FAMILIES
I GREW UP AROUND. STRIVING FOR
EXCELLENCE WAS A GIVEN. NOTHING
WAS TAKEN FOR GRANTED.

....

EMBRACE EXPECTATIONS

I was a kid from Brooklyn, but I went to a high school in Manhattan—an interesting tightrope walk.

The kids in Brooklyn didn't take crap from anybody; they would just as soon get in a fight as play a game of stickball. Then you go into this highly intellectual atmosphere, this high school that's driven by guys in black cassocks called Jesuit priests. It was really a culture change.

There were a lot of people around me who had expectations. In Brooklyn, it was the self-made expectations my mother instilled in me. At school, it was expectations put on me by others: *You're lucky you're here; now you've got to perform.* I really loved it. If you want to excel, what a great place to be in.

PRACTICE COMPASSION

Around 1982 to 1983 I was treating AIDS as a researcher and a physician, but I needed to get out of the lab and find out what I was dealing with. On one trip to New York City, I caught a cab to Greenwich Village to check out the scene.

When I was in high school, we used to go down there, and sometimes go to a bar. I did that in medical school, and I did that as an intern, a resident, a chief resident. We went for the vibrancy of the neighborhood, the incredible spirit of the music, the food, the atmosphere.

My first visit after the advent of HIV was an out-of-body experience, like watching a movie. I already had the experience of taking care of patients with AIDS, some in the very advanced form that we hardly ever see anymore. I walked the streets alone that night and thought, *That guy's got AIDS. That guy's got AIDS. That guy's got AIDS. This guy's got Kaposi sarcoma*. You could see them putting a sweater on—the shiver, the blanches, the purple blotch on their face. What happened to my beautiful Greenwich Village? It had been devastated.

It was a moving but disturbing experience. We weren't in a hospital. We weren't in a laboratory. We were out on the street. It made me appreciate beyond the individual patient, beyond the research of the development of the drugs, what this disease was doing to society.

SACRIFICE FOR THE GREATER GOOD

I cannot figure out this anti-authority, anti-science, anti-mask, anti-anything stance. I get it that we come from the pioneering spirit of our forefathers, the founders of this country. I get all that. But this is taking it to an unreasonable extreme.

It's obvious that wearing a mask is for the good of the public health, and yet it immediately gets turned around that you're encroaching on my civil liberties? It's inherently contradictory. Are your civil liberties encroached on when you wear a seat belt? Or when they tell you that you can't smoke on an airplane? What's the difference?

They're telling you there's an outbreak out there—200,000 cases a day, 2,000 deaths a day, and over 100,000 hospitalizations—and my asking you to wear a mask is encroaching on your civil liberties? I don't understand that. I just don't.

WHEN SOMEONE ASKS ME ABOUT MY EVOLUTION IN WHAT I WANTED TO DO WITH MY LIFE, I ALWAYS SAY IT HAD TO HAVE SOMETHING TO DO WITH DOING THINGS WITH PEOPLE AND FOR PEOPLE.

" IF THE HEALTH OF A COUNTRY IS SIGNIFICANTLY LACKING, IT LEADS TO ECONOMIC INSTABILITY, LEADS TO POLITICAL INSTABILITY, LEADS TO REAL PROBLEMS. PUBLIC HEALTH PERMEATES ALMOST EVERY ASPECT OF OUR LIVES, BOTH DOMESTICALLY AND INTERNATIONALLY.

SCENE
FROM A
LIFE

My sister, Denise, taught me how to dance. As an awkward young teenager, I would go to these dances, since I really wanted to learn how to meet a girl. Denise taught me all the different steps, and I became quite a good dancer as a young person: 12, 13, 14, 15 years old. At the dances, guys would come in from another neighborhood, and it was a lot like the movie *West Side Story* with the Jets and the Sharks. There were quite a number of little rumbles, usually because somebody asked the girl you were dancing with to dance with him instead. That was part of adolescence and growing up on the streets of New York City.

PURSUE YOUR PASSION

3

....

I WAS ALWAYS, AND STILL AM,
VERY SENSITIVE TO PEOPLE WHO
DEVOTE A CONSIDERABLE AMOUNT
OF THEIR LIFE TO SOMETHING.

,

Fauci attended the prestigious Regis High School in Manhattan and went on to study at Holy Cross in Worcester, Massachusetts, then an all-male college. By then, he already knew he wanted to become a doctor.

I n college, I worked every summer in construction as a mason tender, someone who helps a bricklayer (I carried the cement, carried the bricks, cleaned up). I already knew then that I wanted to go to Cornell Medical School, and it was by happenstance that I got picked to work on the construction of the Samuel J. Wood Library at Cornell Medical School, right on York Avenue and East 69th Street in New York City. One day I got up courage to go inside.

When the other construction guys sat down for lunch on the wall, whistling at the nurses going by, I went up the steps and walked in. I looked into the auditorium and remember saying to myself, *Wow, this is amazing.* All of a sudden, the security guard who was standing at the door comes over to me—a big guy. He says, "Can I help you, Sonny?" Sonny. He called me Sonny.

I say, "Oh, I'm just looking around here."

He says, "You got concrete all over your boots. Why don't you just step outside?"

I looked at him, a little bit indignant. I say, "Someday I'm going to be a student in this medical school."

He looked at me with a straight face and he says, "Yes, Sonny. Someday I'm going to be police commissioner of New York City."

A year later, I was a student there.

KEEP YOUR EYES ON THE PRIZE

There wasn't a minute that I didn't treasure in medical school, because it was a phenomenal learning experience day after day after day. My goal was finally getting to see a patient, finally being able to take care of a patient. To me, it was all positive vibrations.

FIND YOUR SOURCE OF JOY AND
EMBRACE IT. AND KEEP THE SOUNDS
OF YOUR LAUGHTER ALIVE.

....

FOLLOW YOUR DREAM

There were certain things immigrant first-generation parents imparted to their second-generation children. You wanted to have a profession: You were a doctor, you were a lawyer, you were an engineer, or you were a priest. (We ruled out priest way back!) I decided that I wanted to become a doctor. One of my sadnesses is that my mother, who really, really would have loved the idea, died when I was in medical school, so she never saw me become a physician.

BE ALL-IN

I loved clinical medicine. The challenge of taking care of a really sick patient was almost, but not quite, intimidating and very, very exciting. Every cell in my body was focused on this: the first time that somebody's life was my responsibility, even though I was only a student. It couldn't get more exciting than that for me.

EVERYTHING COMES BACK TO THE PATIENT. THAT'S A REALLY GOOD FEELING, BECAUSE YOU FEEL ANCHORED IN SOMETHING THAT'S WORTHWHILE.

GET BACK TO BASICS

There are fundamental principles that have guided past generations of physicians—principles that are sometimes forgotten and neglected in the technological world of modern medicine. These are the foundation of the beauty of practicing medicine: integrity, unselfishness, perseverance, inquisitiveness, and a compelling thirst for knowledge.

IF YOU LOOK AT THE HISTORY OF CIVILIZATION—AT SOME OF THE AWFUL THINGS THAT HAVE HAPPENED—YOU WOULD HOPE THAT WE WOULD LEARN TO NEVER REPEAT THEM. WE DO HAVE THE CAPABILITY OF GETTING OFF TRACK AND DOING SOME TERRIBLE THINGS. BUT I AM OPTIMISTIC ABOUT THE FUTURE OF THE HUMAN RACE.

From the time I was born until the time I walked into Regis High School, my name was Anthony. "Anthony, come home." *Anthony, this; Anthony, that.* My friends used to call me Fauch for short.

I walk into my first day at Regis High School, and the dean of discipline at the time—I believe his name was Father Flanagan—said to me, "What's your name?" I replied, "My name is Anthony Fauci." He said, "Tony, welcome to Regis."

Ever since that day, I have been Tony Fauci because everybody heard that Father Flanagan had called me Tony. They'd say, "Hey, Tony, where're you from?" "I'm from Brooklyn." It was *Hey, Tony, this; hey, Tony, that.*

I came home at night and I told my mother and father, "Guess what? My name is Tony now."

They thought that was kind of funny. But my mother liked Anthony. It took her about a decade to get used to Tony. But it was that kind of influence. If the dean of discipline of a Jesuit high school said your name was Tony, your name was Tony. Period. No questions asked.

EXPECT THE UNEXPECTED

4

....

YOU MUST BE PREPARED AT ANY
MOMENT TO ENTER UNCHARTED
TERRITORY, TO EXPECT THE
UNEXPECTED. AND WHERE POSSIBLE,
SEIZE THE OPPORTUNITIES.

,

IN A PANDEMIC, THINGS DON'T GO
AS YOU PLAN, AND YOU HAVE
TO DO A LOT OF IMPROVISATION.
VERY MUCH LIKE IN A WAR.

....

BE READY FOR ANYTHING

Let me give you a personal example of the kinds of dramatic evolutions and changes that can occur totally beyond your control, and that can have a profound impact on the direction of your career and your life.

In 1968, I finished my medical training in internal medicine at New York Hospital–Cornell Medical Center. That same year, noted public health scholars and even the surgeon general were opining and even testifying before the U.S. Congress that with the advent of antibiotics, vaccines, and public health measures, "the war against infectious diseases had been won" and we should focus our efforts on other areas of research and public health.

As fate would have it, at that time I was on my way to begin, of all things, a fellowship for training in infectious diseases at the National Institutes of Health. I remember reflecting as I drove from New York City to the NIH in Bethesda, Maryland, on the words of the wise pundits resonating in my mind, feeling somewhat ambivalent about my career choice, to say the least. Was I entering into a disappearing subspecialty? I sort of felt as if I were going to Miami to become a ski instructor.

But unfortunately and sadly for the world, even surgeons general are not always correct. Indeed, 13 years later, in 1981, the AIDS epidemic had emerged and transformed my professional career, if not my entire life.

YOU HAVE TO LOOSEN UP AND
FIGURE OUT HOW YOU ARE GOING TO
RELATE TO A PERSON'S NEEDS.

. . . .

NO MATTER HOW WELL PREPARED YOU THINK YOU ARE, YOU ARE NOT PREPARED ENOUGH.

....

In 1981, while Fauci was working as one of the leading researchers on immunology and autoimmune diseases at the National Institutes of Health, an as-yet-little-known virus called HIV came onto his radar via an article in the medical journal Morbidity and Mortality Weekly Report, *published by what is now known as the Centers for Disease Control and Prevention. It reported that five gay men from Los Angeles, with no apparent underlying illnesses, had developed a strange pneumonia called pneumocystis pneumonia.*

was sitting in my little office on the 11th floor of the NIH Clinical Center on a hot summer day, the first week in June 1981, when I saw the report. I had been studying drugs that suppressed the immune system, and we were seeing pneumocystis cases. So I thought, *There's something strange going on here,* and put the article in my desk drawer.

One month later, on July 5, another *MMWR* appeared on my desk. This time, 26 men—amazingly, all gay men, and not only from Los Angeles, but from San Francisco and New York—not only had pneumocystis pneumonia, but had Kaposi sarcoma: a tumor, a cancer seen in people whose immune system is dramatically damaged.

I remember looking at that and going, *Oh my God, this is a brand-*

new infectious disease. I actually got goose bumps. I had no idea what the cause of the infection was, but I knew it destroyed the immune system. As a physician-scientist trained in infectious diseases and immunology, if ever there was a disease that was made for me, it was this.

I made a decision then that I was going to completely change the direction of my research. I had been extremely successful in my career, and my mentors, the people who had recruited me here years ago, told me I was crazy. They said, "Why are you throwing away a promising career to go chasing after a disease that's a fluke?" I decided that I was going to do it anyway. I felt obliged to explain it to the world.

Unfortunately, it turned out that I was right. It exploded into one of the most extraordinary pandemics in the history of our civilization.

n 2002, I got a call from one of Bono's inner circle, who said to me, "Bono would love to talk to you about AIDS in Africa."

I say, "Any time your guys are in Washington, just give me a call." He answers, "How about tonight? Do you have a restaurant where you can meet?" I say, "Why don't you just come to my house?"

I live in Northwest D.C. And at the time, my eldest daughter was 13 years old, my middle daughter was 10, and my youngest daughter was seven. So I thought I'd play a trick on my daughter Jenny. I said, "Jen, some guys from my lab are coming over tonight, so if they knock at the door, just let them in."

I'm in my office, and all of a sudden, there's a knock. My daughter goes to the door, and I hear a scream: "Daddy! Bono is here!"

He was wonderful. He spent half an hour just playing with my kids. We cooked a nice pasta and sausage, and he'd brought a couple of terrific bottles of wine. Then we went out on the back deck and were there until the wee hours talking about HIV.

Ever since then, he's been in touch about ways that he can help me and that I can help him. We've actually become good friends.

PERSIST, PERSEVERE, PREVAIL

5

THE MORE ENERGY YOU PUT IN,
THE MORE YOU'RE GOING TO
ACCOMPLISH. IT'S ALMOST INFINITE.

,

ALWAYS PERSEVERE

What I remember most about the early AIDS outbreak is that we were desperately trying to take care of terribly ill and frightened patients who were all young men. Every single day, we came in and worked in the lab, knowing that the patients were so sick. If we ever had a moment to feel badly for ourselves, we would just look at the patients and their families—what they were going through.

In the previous nine years, I had developed a virtually curative therapy for a group of uniformly lethal autoinflammatory diseases. With each new patient, there was a 93 percent chance they were going to walk out of the hospital feeling really good. When I switched over to HIV/AIDS, it was a complete 180-degree turn. I was healing nobody. Nobody.

As much as I tried, I couldn't do anything to prolong their lives. It didn't matter how smart we were because there were no tools. We didn't have a drug for the virus, because at this point we didn't even know what the virus was. We came in every day knowing that we were putting a bandage on a hemorrhage, and that went on not just for months but a few years.

When you get hit with one thing after the other, you've just got to suck it up. I'm grateful for the training I got as a house officer, an intern, and a resident. It laid the foundation of what I can do—and how far I can push myself.

IF THE TIMETABLE DOESN'T WORK,
CHANGE THE TIMETABLE. IF THE
RIGIDITY IS OBSTRUCTIONIST TO
GETTING TO YOUR GOAL, LOOSEN UP.

....

IF AT FIRST YOU DON'T SUCCEED . . .

It's unbelievably frustrating when you're used to being able to fix things, and you're just not fixing anything. That's why it was such a celebration when we finally knew what the virus was. It uplifted all of us doctors at the time. That discovery was transforming: Now I have the virus in my hand, I know what the hell it is; I have it in a test tube. We could begin working on drugs and a vaccine.

The evolution of therapy for HIV is as important a medical advance as any other that I've ever heard of, and that is not hyperbole. We went from an unknown agent that was having almost 100 percent mortality to an agent that had one drug, then two drugs, and then three drugs, and then, essentially, the complete suppression of virus replication to the point where people were starting to live normal lives. Through history, people are going to be talking about how that happened.

"TENS AND TENS AND TENS AND MAYBE HUNDREDS OF MILLIONS OF LIVES HAVE BEEN SAVED BY VACCINES. I BELIEVE WE WILL CRUSH COVID-19. THE VACCINES ARE GOING TO OVERCOME THE PEOPLE WHO DON'T BELIEVE IT'S REAL, WHO SAY IT'S A HOAX AND DON'T WANT TO WEAR A MASK. VACCINES WILL BE THE GREAT EQUALIZER.

NEVER GIVE UP

I'm not afraid of very many things, but what I'm most concerned about is not getting the opportunity to finish the things that I started decades ago, to add the finishing touches.

I would like to see the defining public health challenge of my professional career, HIV, ended as an epidemiological pandemic. Everyone thought we could cure or eradicate AIDS, but that has turned out to be very difficult and could actually be impossible.

I don't think we're going to eradicate HIV—in fact, I know we're not—but I think we can almost eliminate it gradually throughout the world: first in countries that have more resources, but then, ultimately, in sub-Saharan Africa. I would like to be around to see what Hillary Clinton termed "an AIDS-free generation." My fear is that I may not necessarily see that, but I hope I do. And I think I will.

WHEN LIVING THROUGH AN EXTRAORDINARY CHALLENGE AND CRISIS, WE ARE ALL IN IT TOGETHER.

....

M y notoriety—the celebrity aspect of it—is a bit unreal. I'm somewhat uncomfortable with all of the adulation. If you start taking yourself seriously, you get caught up in a whole bunch of ego stuff that's ridiculous.

I find it interesting and amusing, and often run it by my wife, Christine Grady, who's the greatest in the world at putting things into perspective. The thing is, I am more symbolic than real for people. You see people in movies, and you never imagine that you would have any relationship with them, and then they're giving you an award. And on the screen, you see Brad Pitt, Al Pacino, Robert De Niro saying these wonderful things about you. You shake your head and say, *This is nice, but don't get carried away by it, Tony!*

There's a votive candle with my picture on it. I mean, really?

LIVE TO SERVE

6

....

THE CORE OF PUBLIC SERVICE
IS DOING SOMETHING THAT'S
BEYOND YOUR OWN SELF, BEYOND
YOUR OWN POTENTIALLY
SELFISH MOTIVATIONS.

,

SERVE OTHERS

I believe sincerely that regardless of our career paths, we cannot look away from pressing societal issues. There are pockets of society here in our own country that are steeped in poverty, drug abuse, violence, health disparities, inadequate education, discrimination, and despair.

Furthermore, we live in a global society and cannot turn our backs on the terrible and often preventable societal burdens in developing nations: rampant disease, infant mortality, abject poverty in certain regions, starvation, gender inequality, violence against women, and the reappearing specter of genocide.

Public service does not necessarily mean a profession or avocation devoted entirely to service. You can incorporate public service into your life regardless of your chosen career.

WHEN YOU DEVOTE YOUR LIFE
AND YOUR SKILL TO SAVING PEOPLE
FROM SUFFERING AND DEATH,
THAT'S INGRAINED IN YOUR
PERSONALITY AND YOUR DNA.

....

I THINK THE FUNDAMENTAL PRINCIPLES OF GOODNESS AND CARING FOR PEOPLE TRANSCEND RELIGION. THE JESUIT ORDER, WITH ITS PHILOSOPHY OF MEN FOR OTHERS AND THEIR EMPHASIS ON THE INTELLECT AND SERVICE TO OTHERS, HAS HAD MORE INFLUENCE ON ME THAN THE ORGANIZED CHURCH.

BATTLE INEQUITY

In 2000, I went to the Mulago Hospital in Kampala, Uganda, and made rounds with my African colleagues. They presented a case of a young woman who had cryptococcal meningitis and tuberculosis—and who also clearly had AIDS. And they said, "Well, we'll give her treatment for TB and send her home."

I asked, "What about her HIV?" And the doctor answered, "Don't even think about it. We don't have any drugs for HIV." And all of a sudden, it was like, *Holy mackerel, this is me in 1981, '82, '83, making rounds.* The only difference is that we couldn't give patients drugs then because they didn't exist. But this doctor can't treat the patients because he doesn't have the drugs. Back then, we had to watch patients die. But this is 2000!

People were saying that it's Africa; they're not going to be able to take drugs three, four, five times a day. At the time, it was multiple pills multiple times a day for those with AIDS.

That is racism in its absolute clearest form to think that because it's a poor country, a Black country in southern Africa, that you're not able to make use of and benefit from these spectacular scientific discoveries.

I went back home, and that started to eat at me. We had to figure out a way to get some drugs to these people. There was so much inequity there.

WITH THE COVID-19 CRISIS,
WE'RE INVOLVED IN SOMETHING THAT'S
TOTALLY GLOBAL. SO IT'S PUBLIC
SERVICE IN SERVICE OF THE PLANET.

....

MAKE THE WORLD YOUR MISSION

The idea of a public servant hasn't changed in its fundamental meaning for me: What you do is not primarily for yourself but for a greater good than you. That's a core aspect of public service that to me is a very attractive motivation—the idea that you're doing something that is for a purpose that is positive for the world in general or for individuals within the world. It makes me feel good about what I do.

Identifying an effective cocktail of antiretroviral drugs transformed the lives of people living with HIV/AIDS. But because more than 90 percent of infections occurred in resource-limited countries where the lifesaving drugs were inaccessible, President George W. Bush tasked Fauci in 2002 with designing a program to address the humanitarian crisis. The resulting plan, the President's Emergency Plan for AIDS Relief (PEPFAR), is credited with dramatically slowing the spread of the disease across the globe, building health care capacity in 50 countries, and saving over 20 million lives.

eorge W. Bush has a strong spirit of empathy and social responsibility. He's a compassionate guy who really, really cared about our moral responsibility to make sure that there are not people in the world who are dying of a disease (AIDS) that we have control over.

Getting awarded the Presidential Medal of Freedom from Bush was one of the most extraordinarily positive experiences that I've ever had, for a number of reasons: the president who gave it to me, the context in which it was given, and what I had done up to that point to actually deserve it. I received the Medal of Freedom fundamentally for being one of the primary architects of PEPFAR. It was President George W. Bush's vision: He was the one who sent me to Africa for feasibility studies, the one who listened to me when I came back. To have him bestow on me the highest honor for a civilian in the United States, to have somebody like that put the medal around my neck for something he and I were partners on, was beyond extra special.

"WHEN I HEAR THE STRESS AND THE STRAIN OF THE PEOPLE IN THE EMERGENCY ROOMS AND INTENSIVE CARE UNITS TREATING COVID-19, I KNOW ABSOLUTELY WHAT THEY'RE GOING THROUGH, BECAUSE I'VE BEEN THERE. AND THEY DO IT EVERY SINGLE DAY, DAY AFTER DAY, WEEK AFTER WEEK, MONTHS IN A ROW. I HAVE SUCH ADMIRATION FOR THEM.

On a beautiful, crisp, sunny morning in 2020, Christine and I went down to a space adjacent to RFK Stadium in Washington, D.C. An artist, Suzanne Brennan Firstenberg, had done something breathtaking: She had covered acres with hundreds of thousands of little white flags stuck in the ground, representing each person who had died from COVID-19—about 250,000 at the time.

It makes viewers realize two things—first, the total enormity of the burden of suffering and death, and second, because they were individual flags, it just blasted that these are individual human beings with a mother, a father, a sister, a brother, a husband, a wife. The contrast of the sun rising in a crystal-clear sky and then this sea of flags was an extraordinarily moving experience. Walking through, we noticed that some people had written the name, date of birth, and date of death of the people whom those flags represented.

We knew a young man, Christopher—an otherwise healthy 32-year-old, the brother of my daughter's boyfriend—who got COVID and died within two weeks of becoming ill. It was really tough to accept. Chris wrote Christopher's name on a flag and put the flag in the ground.

LEAD BY EXAMPLE

7

LEADERSHIP TAKES MANY
FORMS, INCLUDING THE QUIET
AND SUBTLE LEADERSHIP
OF EXAMPLE.

,

DON'T FOR A MOMENT BELIEVE
THAT YOU ARE TOO YOUNG OR TOO
INEXPERIENCED TO BEGIN TO ASSUME
LEADERSHIP ROLES. YOU DO NOT
NEED TO WAIT.

....

STEP UP

Somebody had to step up to the plate to be a leader in not only the national but also the global fight against the historic COVID-19 pandemic. I felt I had to take on responsibilities that were not part of my job description, ones that people in my job had never assumed. Somebody had to do it. There had to be a national movement toward going to the next level.

SPEAK UP

I liked Ronald Reagan. I thought he was a good person, but he did not pay the kind of attention he should have to HIV/AIDS. Reagan did not use the bully pulpit of the presidency during his first term to call attention to the emerging AIDS outbreak. If he had said, "Hey, everybody! This could be a real problem," he could have made a difference. People might have been alerted to the real, devastating potential of this outbreak.

There was a reticence in the Reagan administration to speak openly about this disease. To the great dismay of the people who liked him, Reagan never uttered the word "AIDS" until his second term, when Elizabeth Taylor essentially forced him to talk about it at a meeting that I was at. Good for Elizabeth.

Reagan was a president who missed the opportunity by omission. That's similar to the Trump administration: For COVID-19, Trump didn't use the bully pulpit of the presidency and the Oval Office and the White House press room to sound the alarm about the seriousness of this crisis. In fact, what happened was worse than with Reagan. Reagan never said "Don't worry about it"; he just ignored it. Trump, on the other hand, underplayed the seriousness of COVID-19.

With all of Reagan's good qualities, when it came to HIV, his legacy is going to be that he did not use the powers of the presidency.

CLARITY MATTERS

You've got to have one sharp, clear message. When you try to have two or three or four messages, your audience will remember *no* messages. What's most important is to have precision of thought and economy of expression. Don't be scatterbrained. Focus on your message, define the problem, and articulate it in as few words and as clearly as possible.

WHEN YOU'RE DEALING WITH THE
RESPONSIBILITY FOR PEOPLE'S
HEALTH AND THEIR LIVES, YOU NEED
A STRONG MORAL COMPASS.

....

KNOW YOUR AUDIENCE

Don't speak to the American public as you would to the National Academy of Sciences, and don't speak to the National Academy of Sciences as you would to a sixth-grade class. And when you're speaking to the public on a subject that they don't intuitively understand, don't try to show them how smart you are. If you put something in an arcane, convoluted way to an audience of 100, one or two people will think you're brilliant, and 98 or 99 won't have a clue what you're talking about. You may take great gratification and think you're incredibly smart, but you'll be completely ineffective in getting your message across.

KEEP YOUR COOL

Sometimes you have to show righteous indignation, but don't let it get out of control. Be patient. Don't ever be hostile with anybody—although if they out-and-out insult you, you have to show that you're not going to stand for that. I use *The Godfather* as the great book of philosophy: It's nothing personal, strictly business. Don't get into the fray, don't get defensive, and don't play into the bait that's being thrown your way.

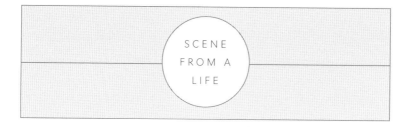

've testified before Congress several hundred times—for better or worse, more than anybody else, ever. When I go there, I'm representing NIH, the Department of Health and Human Services, and, in many respects, the administration.

To act as one branch of government interacting with another is both exciting and fun, because the branch that you're testifying before is checking on you. That's their job. I like the idea that they have the right to ask me any question they want, and being under oath adds a little special punch to it.

I would say that 99 percent of the times that I've testified before Congress, it was either on C-SPAN or live-streamed on CNN, so the public knew what was going on. There's a certain purity about that, a reflection of democracy. There it is: the government laid bare right in front of you. Nothing is covered up.

I was born and raised on the streets of New York, but I'm a creature of Washington. Over the 50 years I've been here, I've grown to love the institutions and how they work, to love the executive branch of which I'm a part, to love what the legislative branch can do. It's extraordinary.

BE A
LIFELONG
LEARNER

8

. . . .

THE MOSAIC OF YOUR
KNOWLEDGE AND EXPERIENCES
IS ETERNALLY UNFINISHED,
AS IT SHOULD BE.

,

Fauci's work at NIH made him uniquely prepared to face the coronavirus epidemic. He had already worked on treatment and prevention—and importantly, vaccine development—for the Zika virus, Ebola, anthrax, pandemic flu, HIV, tuberculosis, and other diseases. But he's acutely aware of the public's short memory: We say we learn from experience, but how can we make sure that's really true?

think that when you get further and further away from a profoundly defining event, the impact of that attenuates. In 1918 during the Spanish flu pandemic, my father was eight years old. I'm sure the horror of that year and a half influenced him as he moved into his teenage years and his 20s and 30s. And then it probably diminished, but he never forgot it.

For those of us like me who only read about it as a vague story in a history book, it doesn't have the same impact of being there or being intimately connected with someone who experienced it.

I think it's the same thing you see in every aspect of those who witnessed the devastation of the early years of HIV. When you were there and you had no tools, you had no idea what the disease was, and all of these really nice young gay men were dying. Fast-forward 35 years, and there is no way that a physician who has never seen that can really appreciate what that was like. You can tell that person about it and explain it, but it's not the same.

I was born in 1940. World War II ended when I was almost five years old. The people who came back from the war and the experience they had could never be translated to people 40 years later: What do you mean you were in a place where you invaded an island and 10,000 of your friends got killed?

I don't think not understanding is a failing; it's just the way life is. Unless you're connected with something directly, it doesn't mean much to you. The COVID-19 epidemic is not like anything else we have experienced in the past 102 years. Let us not forget that we were not as prepared as we thought we were or as we should have been. So let's get to being able to say, "Never again. We're never going to let this happen again."

What I'm afraid of as we get out of this is that it's going to be five years from now, 10 years from now, and people are just going to either forget or not care how this outbreak completely gripped the world. They're going to forget.

I say this with a bit of despair: that we've always been aware of health disparities. We're always aware that African American and Hispanic people get the short end of the stick with disease, and their disproportionate burden with COVID-19 now is staring us right in the face.

Let us make a commitment that in the next three or four decades, we're going to do something about that. Sounds great. But five years from now, some other problem is going to come along, and we're going to forget about COVID-19.

LIVE TO LEARN

The consequences of getting something wrong can be serious to a young physician and scientist; in fact, this is true to a greater or lesser degree in any chosen career path. It is this feeling, this tension, that can serve as the catalyst to constantly improve yourself, and this will be counterbalanced by the palpable excitement of continual learning. After all these years, I still derive energy and motivation from that very subtle tension, and I still marvel at how much fun the learning process is.

IN WHATEVER FIELD OR CAREER PATH
YOU CHOOSE, IF YOU ARE TO BE TRUE
TO YOURSELF AND LIVE UP TO YOUR
FULL POTENTIAL, YOU WILL LIVE
YOUR LIFE AS A PERPETUAL STUDENT.

....

'YOU'VE GOT TO BE
HUMBLE ENOUGH, AND
MODEST ENOUGH, AND KNOW
THAT YOU HAVE TO KEEP
LEARNING. I AM NOW
A PRETTY OLD GUY, AND
YET EVERY DAY, I'M
LOOKING THINGS UP THAT
I DON'T KNOW, OR I
NEED TO BE REMINDED OF.

YOU WILL NEVER KNOW AS MUCH AS
YOU WANT TO OR NEED TO KNOW,
AND YOU WILL FIND THAT YOU ARE
PARTICIPATING IN A DYNAMIC PROCESS
WITH A STEEP LEARNING CURVE.
YOU CAN'T BE IMMOBILIZED.

....

DETAILS MATTER

I am, as I always say, nonpathologically obsessive compulsive, which I think works well for me. Rather than causing me stress, it actually relieves me when I know everything's exactly the way I want it to be.

As a resident in medicine, even when I was very tired, I would check the gauges on every one of the respirators on every one of the IVs in the ICU before I went to bed, making sure that they were all flowing. You have to check everything; you can't just assume that it's going to be okay. And in the long run, these details aren't really adding time; they're saving you time.

KEEP CURRENT

Because medicine and its related disciplines are based on fundamental and immutable principles, I did not fully appreciate how dramatically the biological sciences and my chosen field would change. You have one foot in the medical past as you take gigantic leaps into the medical future. Rest assured that being bored is not a problem.

I continue to be both exhilarated and a little bit intimidated as science advances at a breathtaking pace. The excitement that still grips me after all these years is from being a part of that evolution—even if it means hanging on for dear life just to keep up.

YOU HAVE TO BE EXCELLENT,
AND THEN YOU WORK YOUR WAY
UP FROM EXCELLENT.

....

When my family moved from Bensonhurst, the nuns in school, Our Lady of Guadalupe, didn't want to lose me because I was, they said, "the smartest kid in the class." We used to have citywide spelling bees, and they figured if they could keep me in the class, they'd have a good chance of winning.

I remember it was at an auditorium in downtown Brooklyn, and I did really well. The 17th round, 16th, 15th, 14th. We got down to the third or the fourth round, and they asked me to spell the word "millennium." And I spelled it "M-I-L-E-N-I-U-M."

"Wrong, Anthony. You're out."

The teachers forgave me, and they were rewarded by the fact that I became the first person from our school to get into Regis High School, which to them was a big thing. So it paid off.

And now there's no chance in the world I'll ever misspell the word *millennium*.

FORGE

PARTNERSHIPS

9

....

WE LIVE IN A GLOBAL COMMUNITY.
THAT MEANS INTERCONNECTIVITY.
THAT MEANS COMMUNICATION.
THAT MEANS TRANSPARENCY.

,

While treatments for HIV/AIDS evolved inside scientific laboratories, frustrated activists demanding equitable access to new antiretroviral drugs and greater representation in clinical trials were vocally critical of Fauci and his NIH team, even picketing their office. Most of Fauci's peers refused to engage with the community, reasoning that emotion had no place in science. Yet Fauci invited the activists in for a conference and began building bridges between the community and lab, eventually forming a deep friendship with his former antagonist, Larry Kramer, the founder of ACT UP.

My first evidence that there was anger at the government's response to the HIV crisis was when it became clear that I, who had been knocking myself out trying to do the right thing, was the object of anger—in the form of, most prominently, a man named Larry Kramer, who was a firebrand activist. In the modern history of medicine, there's before Larry Kramer and after Larry Kramer. Larry was the godfather and initiator of the AIDS activist movement, the person who screamed out with passion that we needed to do something. And that's what we needed: the jolt. The activist community shook the cages.

Instead of reacting, I focused on the pain and fear that prompted their confrontational approach. I put aside the theatrics and listened to what the activists were saying. And when the noise got out of the way, it became patently clear to me that they were making absolute sense. If we're not strong enough to deal with diverse opinions from activists, then we're not worth it.

STRIVE FOR UNDERSTANDING

Activists are mistaken when they assume that scientists do not care about them. Most scientists care deeply and are employing all of their energies and talents to accomplish the same goal as the activists are. By the same token, scientists cannot and should not dismiss activists merely because they are not trained scientists. Scientists do not need to adhere to every suggestion made by activists because some of them may be misguided. However, scientists themselves do not have a lock on correctness.

We must join together, for together we are a formidable force with a common goal.

IN THE FIELD THAT I'M IN, GETTING PUBLIC SUPPORT IS ABSOLUTELY CRITICAL BECAUSE IT'S IMPORTANT FOR PEOPLE GETTING VACCINATED—AND FOR PEOPLE TO ACCEPT AND SUPPORT SCIENCE.

....

TRUST YOUR TEAM

When you have a really, really sick patient, you are almost never in the room alone with that patient. You have nurses, doctors, respiratory therapists, and others there consulting. It's almost like a tight basketball game where everybody has got to be on their game or you're going to lose.

With basketball, you're always relying on somebody else. Somebody's got to give you the ball, and you've got to pass it back. You have to play defense. You have to play offense. And what is particularly good is when the team hums well together.

That doesn't happen in every game. It doesn't happen every play, but there's something about a good, fast break. Somebody grabs the rebound, flips it to the guy on the side, hits it to the guy in the middle, a couple of dribbles, fake one way, boom, layup that's in. That's like music or art when that happens.

OPEN LINES OF COMMUNICATION

When in Washington, be nice to everybody, because you never know where they're going to wind up.

When George H. W. Bush was vice president, he saw that HIV/AIDS was an important issue, and as part of his plan to run for president, he felt that he needed to learn more. So he came to the NIH, and I spent hours with him. That's unusual. When presidents visit, you usually spend 10 or 15 minutes.

I showed him the wards where we were making rounds. He thanked me profusely and wrote me a thank-you note. And then he became my friend. He would invite my wife, Christine, and me to brunches and dinners at the vice president's mansion. He would call me with questions. He didn't go through the secretary or the assistant secretary. He just called.

He promised me that if he became president of the United States, one of the first things he would do is come back and visit me again at the NIH and that he would do what he could to increase our budget. And sure enough, he became president of the United States, and our funding went way up.

He was one of the most attentive people imaginable. I would be in the news, and I would get a handwritten note afterward saying, "Tony, saw you on TV last night. You're looking good! What are you doing to look so fit?"

n the early '80s, I was buried in my work. One day I had a patient who spoke only Portuguese, so they called in a nurse, Christine Grady, to translate. I looked at her and thought, *Wow, who's this?*

Now, Chris will tell you (though I deny this) that everybody was afraid of me. I'm not a mean person, but I demand excellence. Chris had heard that I was this scary guy, so she was nervous.

She translated for the patient: "He wants to go back to Rio de Janeiro, where he lives." I said, "Okay, but he needs to keep his legs elevated and change the dressings frequently. If he does that, I'll let him go."

She spoke to the patient; he talked back. As it turned out, he said, "I've been sitting in this bed for a month and a half. When I go back to Rio, I'm going to go out drinking and dancing." So Chris made a judgment call and said, "He's going to do exactly as you say."

A few days later, I said to myself that I really needed to figure out who this person was. I told one of the nurses to send her to my office. Chris was mortified, figuring that I'd found out she'd lied. She sat down, and I said, "Would you like to go to dinner?" Her jaw dropped.

She moved in that May, and we married the following May.

REVERE THE TRUTH

10

......

IF YOU REALLY WANT TO BE
EFFECTIVE, YOU'VE GOT TO ALWAYS
KNOW THAT YOU'RE GOING TO
TELL THE TRUTH, EVEN THOUGH IT
MAY BE SOMETHING THAT SOMEONE
DOESN'T WANT TO HEAR.

,

Fauci was appointed to President Trump's White House Coronavirus Task Force, created in early 2020 to address the COVID-19 pandemic. He became a frequent, if unofficial, spokesman for the White House during the pandemic, appearing regularly on television and radio to update the public and advocate for public health measures like social distancing and mask wearing.

D onald J. Trump and I kind of liked each other. Maybe it was the "having New York in common" thing. This was my sixth administration. We developed, as I think both of us have described, an interesting relationship, a good one. But more than once, as we would get into the press conferences, I would have to fine-tune something that he said. That seemed to be surprisingly okay until things started to get a bit more tense. And yet when I would see him two days later in the Oval Office, it was as if we were buddies again. I don't think he had a deliberate, malicious disdain for science. I think he just didn't think it was important. It's not even disdain; it's a disregard.

I was not surprised when President Trump contracted COVID— not that I wished him any ill; in some respects I like the guy. He was the president of the United States, and I have the utmost respect for the office of the presidency. I didn't want to see anything bad happen to him, but when I was asked, I said I wasn't surprised because he was behaving in a way that was absolutely conducive to getting infected.

When it was clear that some of the things that he was saying were contradictory to the scientific facts, I became uncomfortable standing there on the stage, giving an implicit ratification of what he was saying.

I felt my job was to do whatever I could to get us out of this outbreak, so leaving my position was not an option. The only option I had was to take the chance, right in that venue, to contradict him. I could either keep quiet, which would be violating my own principles, or leave, which would have meant I wouldn't be able to do any more good. I felt the only way I could maintain scientific integrity was to speak up.

It was clear that my message to the American public was contrary to his message, so he allowed the legions around him to try to undermine my credibility. Yet he had this interesting, complicated relationship with me, and I don't think he wanted to hurt me. I think he was torn by the fact that, deep down, he knew that what I was saying was true. He liked me, but what I was saying was unacceptable to him.

BELIEVE IN YOURSELF

I have worked with seven presidents over the course of 11 terms. I learned from the very beginning that you're doomed to failure if you are afraid of not getting asked back, if you're afraid of saying something that's going to get somebody upset. Nobody wants the president of the United States to be upset with you.

During the Trump administration, every once in a while I would say something that the administration didn't like, and then I would be off television for a week or so. But I would always come back. I didn't want to lose that. I didn't want to lose the direct messaging to the American public.

STAND BY YOUR CONVICTIONS

My wife, Christine, has taught me a number of things. I think I have a strong moral compass, but it is extraordinary living with someone who is really brave in standing by her convictions, who has the highest degree of integrity and ethics. She lives by that, and she teaches me that I can even be better than I am now.

THE BEST ROUTE TO TRUTH IS SCIENCE,
PHILOSOPHY, ART—ALL OF THE ABOVE. FOR ME,
SCIENCE COMES FIRST, BUT I GOT TO WHERE
I AM THROUGH UNDERSTANDING THE HUMAN
SPIRIT.

....

ACCEPT REALITY

One of the things that still completely baffles me is the lack of acceptance by some people in this country that COVID is a problem. There are people who think that this is a hoax, some made-up thing for one reason or other, when the facts are staring us right in the face. That tells me that we have some fundamental lesions in this country that need to be addressed and healed. I know that people who are feeling that way are looking at me and saying I'm the crazy one. But I'm sorry, I have to call you on this: It's crazy to think that this is not real.

ABOUT ANTHONY FAUCI

Anthony Fauci is one of the most celebrated doctors in the world. Born in New York City in 1940, he grew up in an Italian American immigrant neighborhood of Brooklyn attending parochial schools until earning a place at the competitive Regis High School in Manhattan. In 1966 he graduated Cornell Medical College. He served as a clinical associate at the National Institutes of Health before making a legendary run as chief resident at New York Hospital. Throughout his long career in clinical research and public service, Fauci maintains that his primary identity is as a physician.

In 1981 Fauci began researching a new epidemic that eventually would be identified as HIV/AIDS. His lab pioneered lifesaving treatments for the disease, and he became a lead architect on PEPFAR, a program that disseminated them around the world. Appointed director of the National Institute of Allergy and Infectious Diseases in 1984, he has advised every president since Ronald Reagan, frequently testifies before Congress, and has responded to outbreaks of anthrax, Ebola, H1N1, and SARS. At the onset of the 2020 COVID-19 pandemic, Fauci helped oversee the development of an effective vaccine within a year.

Anthony Fauci is the recipient of numerous awards, including the Presidential Medal of Freedom and the National Medal of Science. The father of three daughters, he lives with his wife, Christine, in Washington, D.C.

"IF HISTORIANS LOOK BACK AT WHAT I'VE DONE IN MY LIFE, I HOPE THEY SEE A LIFE OF COMMITMENT TO HAVING A POSITIVE IMPACT ON SOCIETY. AND I HAVE HAD SOME DEGREE OF SUCCESS IN DOING SO. MAYBE SOMEBODY MANY, MANY YEARS FROM NOW GOES BACK AND READS ABOUT THIS AND SAYS, HEY, THAT GUY WAS PRETTY GOOD.